Publis

MW01610688

@ Levi Perry

Ketogenic Diet: Amazing Health and Delicious

Ketogenic Diet Recipes

Weights Loss and Healthy Life

All Right RESERVED

ISBN 978-1-990053-91-7

TABLE OF CONTENTS

Chapter 1 1

What Is A Keto Diet? 1

Chapter 2 How To Maximize Fat Loss 5

Chapter 3 9

More Things That You Need To Know 9

Chapter 4 17

Low Carb High-Fat Keto Recipes 17

Vanilla Chai Smoothie 17

Cinnamon Almond Porridge 19

Coco-Cashew Macadamia Muffins 21

Chocolate Protein Pancakes 23

Chive, Cheddar, Ham, And Omelet 25

Spinach Parmesan Egg Scramble 27

Eggs And Russet Potatoes 29

Turkey Chili 31

Almond Chicken Breast Saute 33

Almond Cod Fish And Spinach 35

Habanero And Bell Pepper Soup................................. 38

Squash And Red Lentil.. 40

Chapter 5.. 42

Breakfast Recipes 42

Eggs And Sausage Breakfast Casserole 42

Sausage Quiche 44

Mini Eggs In Cups 46

Breakfast Skillet.. 48

Blueberry Pancakes.. 50

Chorizo And Cauliflower Breakfast 51

Bacon Avocado Breakfast Tacos 53

Chive, Bacon, And Cheddar Omelet........................... 55

Egg Cups 57

Cinnamon Roll Oatmeal 59

Chive, Cheddar, And Ham Soufflé 61

Spinach Omelet.. 63

Cheese And Sausage Breakfast Pie 65

Egg Baskets.. 67

Chapter 6... 69

Keto Salad Recipes 69

Mixed Green Spring Salad 69

Pork Salad.. 70

Caprese Salad 72

Cucumber Salad 73

Spinach Salad 75

Egg Salad 76

Chapter 7... 78

Keto Main Dish Recipes... 78

Mandarin Chicken W/ Homemade Orange Sauce 78

Ginger + Coconut-Spiced Chicken 80

Turkey Gravy 82

Cheesy Turkey "Pasta" 84

Turkey-Stuffed Bell Peppers....................................... 86

Beef Bourguignon 88

Easiest Short Ribs 90

Slow-Cooker Swiss Steak Veggies 91

Cider-Braised Beef Shank 92

Coconut-Ginger Beef 94

Classic Pot Roast... 95

Italian-Style Pot Roast 97

Cinnamon Roll Waffles 99

Bacon Swiss Waffles 101

Spinach Cauliflower Soup 103

Cheesy Buffalo Chicken Sandwich 105

Coconut Chicken Tenders 107

Avocado Spinach Salad With Almonds 109

Easy Chopped Salad 110

Cauliflower Leek Soup With Pancetta 111

Three Meat And Cheese Sandwich 113

Chicken Caesar Salad Wrap 115

Spiced Carrot Ginger Soup 117

Seared Salmon With Baby Arugula 119

Goat Cheese And Bell Pepper Salad........................ 121

Fusil Salad... 122

Cream Cheese Chive Omelet.................................... 124

Spanish Omelet 125

Spinach And Mushroom Omelet.............................. 126

Keto Bacon And Egg Casserole................................ 127

Mexican Breakfast.. 129

Keto Smoothie.. 131

Coconut Porridge 132

Donuts 134

Keto Blueberry Smoothie 136

Slow Cooker Pizza... 137

Holiday Lamb W/ Mint + Asparagus 138

Spinach-Lamb Curry 140

Easy Shredded Taco Pork 141

Pork Adobo Tacos 142

Ribs Homemade Sauce............................. 145

Pork Shoulder Gravy 147

Mustard-Glazed Ham 149

Rum-Glazed Ham 150

Chapter 1

What Is A Keto Diet?

The ketogenic diet is a low-carb, moderate-protein, and high-fat diet. Unlike other diets, the keto diet forces the body to use different fuel sources for energy. Usually, the body relies on carb (sugar) reserves as fuel. When following a normal carb-rich diet, the cells, tissues, and organs use up glucose from carbohydrates and convert it into energy. While this is the ideal biochemistry for the body, consuming too many carbs leads to an excess of glucose in the blood. If the cells are no longer able to use the excess, it gets stored in the liver as glycogen and eventually converted into fats. This means that if your physical activity is too little, you end up accumulating fat in your body, leading to chronic problems such as high blood pressure, obesity, diabetes, and others.

How Keto Works

The Keto diet focuses on the drastic reduction of carbohydrates and replaces these carbs with fats. When you follow the keto diet, your body bypasses glucose and instead uses fats as its main fuel source. When the body detects little carbohydrates in the bloodstream, it automatically turns on another pathway that burns the stored fat into energy.

This is when the body enters into a state called ketosis. Ketosis is the ultimate goal of the keto diet. Ketosis is a metabolic process where the body is forced to use body fat for energy instead of carbs and sugars.

Entering Ketosis

You need to understand ketosis to understand the ketogenic diet. Ketosis is a process whereby the body burns off fat as an alternative energy source in the absence or deficit of glucose. Under normal circumstances, the body uses the hormone glucose to push glucose into cells to provide energy. Low glucose levels switch on another metabolic pathway in the body, which is ketosis, to burn off fats as an energy source. Ketosis is a normal process, and it plays a vital role in humans' evolutionary success.

With keto, your body starts to use fat as fuel. Once your body has limited access to blood glucose or sugar, your body will enter a state of ketosis. With keto, the levels of insulin hormones in your body decrease, and the fatty acids in your body will be released from the fat stores.

From this point, the fatty acids that are being released into your body are then transferred to your liver. Once in place, the fatty acids are oxidized and turned into ketone bodies, which provide your body with energy. Once the process has occurred, ketones provide energy for your body and your brain without ever needing glucose.

Chapter 2

How To Maximize Fat Loss

There is no doubt that you will lose weight the first week you start doing the ketogenic diet. It's almost foolproof. I see average Joes and average Janes of all ages losing weight and looking great just by eating a ketogenic diet. But this is where everyone falls short. They just rely on the diet to achieve their physical goals or their definition of fitness. Let me explain to you how you can maximize your fat loss by incorporating keto into your lifestyle.

The first thing you should be doing is pretty obvious. You should be working out. The great thing about being in a state of ketosis is that you are using fat for energy. People who don't work out are just burning fat for everyday activities like walking at work and sustaining their lifestyle. In other words, they are losing weight while being sedentary. This is a terrible way to take advantage of being in ketosis. Instead, you should participate in some form of exercise to hit the gas pedal on that fat-burning state you are in. I like to think of it this way. If a person that wasn't in ketosis went on a treadmill for an hour then they will lose 1 pound. But a person in ketosis on a treadmill for an hour will lose 5 pounds. Again, that's just a theoretical example of how it's much more efficient to work out in a ketosis state than not. Besides working out or movement of your body is needed. You were made to move, and our bodies getting stronger and living longer by doing so. We were not meant to be sedentary! So whether you are doing the ketogenic lifestyle or not you should start developing some form of exercise in your daily or weekly routine.

Here is a hack that can put your ketosis fat-burning power into overdrive! Another very popular fitness and health hack is intermittent fasting. Intermittent fasting is a style of eating where you have a period of being fast, usually 12-16 hours, and a window of eating for the rest of the day. I remember when I first heard of it. I thought it was so extreme! Seeing the transformations and discipline that one had, to go hours without eating was amazing. The period of being fasted looked like it was worth it to have an amazing transformation. One of the main goals of intermittent fasting is to put the body in mild ketosis and induce autophagy. Autophagy is the breakdown of old cells and creating stronger new ones. I strongly suggest doing more research on autophagy if you are into anti-aging. So here's the hack, do intermittent fasting and keto at the same time! Simply have a period of being fasted 12-16 hours and eat your allowance of calories in the remaining hours of the day. Being fasting will put you in ketosis and put you in a state where you burn more fat because you didn't consume any calories to burn. When you eat your ketogenic meal you will still stay in ketosis. But the times you have fasted your fat burning will be much more than just doing keto alone. I remember when I first tried this, the weight came off tremendously. And now 16-20 hours of being fast is a piece of cake. No pun intended. Simply put keto and intermittent fasting are great ways of increasing your health and losing weight. Putting both diets together is like magnifying your results in a shorter time.

Chapter 3

More Things That You Need To Know

How will I benefit from the Keto diet?

 One great thing about this diet is that it will help reduce your appetite. People end up cheating while dieting due to a simple reason: they're hungry. But when you adhere to the keto diet plan, your appetite will naturally diminish. This way, it becomes easier for you to stick to the program in the long run.

For most people, fat is fat, whether the stuff is deposited in your arms, your thighs, or your tummy. What they don't understand is that the fat's *location* in the body is equally serious as its presence. One reason that sets the keto diet apart from other reducing diets is that it helps get rid of fat in the proper places. The fat seated in your abdominal cavity and surrounding your vital organs is visceral fat that puts you in danger of suffering from metabolic conditions and inflammatory diseases. Thankfully, a great portion of the fat that is lost when adhering to the keto diet is the fats lodged in the abdominal region.

Unlike high carbohydrate diets, keto diets are more effective in lowering your risk of developing a cardiac disease. That's because this diet limits the presence of triglycerides (fat molecules) in your bloodstream. The keto diet also increases the levels of good cholesterol in your blood.

Carb-rich diets change the pH in your mouth, making you predisposed to developing dental diseases. Conversely, the keto diet improves your teeth and gum health in just a few months.

Another advantage of adhering to this diet is that you'll experience less bloating. Gas pains are common in high-carb diets, which are chock-full of sugars and grains. These irritants are eliminated in keto diet plans.

The ketogenic diet prevents inflammatory health conditions by reducing the amount of C Reactive Protein in your system. People with chronic joint problems also report experiencing less pain after switching to the keto diet.

High-carb diets consisting of too many grains cause some people to suffer from gastroesophageal reflux disease. When you follow the keto diet, you can exclude grain-based sources.

When you adhere to the low-carb, high-fat diet plan, you'll notice immediate changes. High carb meals tend to make your head feel foggy. Conversely, keto diet meals allow your brain to function in optimum capacity.

This diet also helps in balancing the levels of dopamine and serotonin in your system resulting in more stable moods.

When you eat high-carb meals, you tend to feel sleepy in the afternoon. This ends up disturbing your sleeping pattern. On the other hand, a low-carb, high-fat meal ensures that you are full of energy throughout the day. You get to think, you become more productive, and you feel a general sense of wellness.

What side effects should I expect as I begin switching to the keto diet?

In the beginning, you'll experience frequent urination. This occurs as glycogen is broken down and forms large amounts of water as a byproduct. However, this will only occur during the first week or perhaps a few more days after that. The solution? Drink plenty of water to replace what you've lost.

Water is not the only thing that you'll lose during those recurrent trips to the bathroom. Your kidneys will also be eliminating sodium, magnesium, and potassium. As a result, you might experience a bit of headache, dizziness, fatigue, or muscle cramps. When this occurs, make sure that you include 5 mg of salt in your daily diet. Add more potassium-rich foods to your meals. Adding two cups of leafy greens to your daily meals will make up for the loss. With your physician's approval, you can take Mg Citrate at night as a supplement.

Another side effect associated with water loss is constipation. However, you can avoid this problem once you replace the lost fluid and correct sodium and magnesium imbalances by adjusting your diet. If not, the solution would be to lessen your consumption of dairy.

Some individuals may experience diarrhea during the first few days. The usually occurs when you don't eat enough fats and consume more protein than you should. A solution would be to take one teaspoon of psyllium husk before eating a meal.

Beware of eating too much lean protein and too little fats. This will cause an alteration in your metabolic processes resulting in a condition known as "rabbit starvation". When this happens, you'll feel hungry all the time and thus, you'll end up consuming more food and gaining more weight than you should.

It's normal to experience transient hypoglycemia during the transition period. Your body has gotten so used to the high-carb diet that it has also gotten used to releasing levels of insulin to match all that sugar. A sudden switch will lead to *temporary* hypoglycemic episodes. To prevent this, begin your transition to the keto lifestyle with small, frequent meals.

It is important to understand that all these side effects are manageable and sometimes even completely avoidable. In any case, they are certainly not life-threatening. Moreover, you can expect these symptoms to disappear once you get used to the keto state.

The ketogenic diet is suitable for everyone except those who are suffering from metabolic illnesses, liver diseases, renal failure, pancreatitis, and diseases of the gall bladder. Individuals who have had gastric bypass surgery are not candidates for following this diet.

As this diet works by using fat as a substitute source of energy, people with conditions that prevent them from digesting fat normally are not advised to try this diet. Other poor candidates for the keto diet include those who suffer from malnutrition and those with cases of long-chain acyl dehydrogenase and pyruvate carboxylase deficiencies.

Chapter 4

Low Carb High-Fat Keto Recipes

Vanilla Chai Smoothie

Ingredients:

- 1/2 tsp. of ground ginger
- Liquid stevia
- Pinch ground cardamom
- 1 cup of plain full-fat yogurt
- 1 cup of unsweetened almond milk
- 1 tsp. of vanilla extract
- 1/2 tsp. of ground cinnamon
- Pinch ground cloves

Preparations:

1. Include every one of the Ingredients: inside a blender.

2. For several times, pulse the ingredient and then blend until it becomes smooth.
3. Dispense inside a large glass and serve.

Cinnamon Almond Porridge

Ingredients:

- 1/4 tsp. of ground cinnamon
- 1 tbsp. of almond butter
- 1/2 cup of canned coconut milk
- Pinch salt
- 1 tbsp. of coconut flour
- 1 tbsp. of butter
- 1 whisked large egg

Preparations:

1. Under low heat in a saucepan, melt the butter.
2. Whisk the egg, coconut flour, salt, and cinnamon in.
3. While whisking, include the coconut milk and then add the almond butter.
4. Thorough stir so that it becomes smooth.

5. On low heat, simmer, and keep stirring frequently until everything is thoroughly heated.
6. Spoon the desired quantity into a bowl, serve and enjoy!

Coco-Cashew Macadamia Muffins

Ingredients:

- 1/2 tsp. of salt

- 2 cups of melted cashew butter

- 2 cups of unsweetened almond milk

- 4 large eggs

- 1 cup of powdered erythritol

- 1/2 cup of chopped macadamia nuts

- 2 cups of almond flour

- 1/2 cup of unsweetened cocoa powder

- 2 tsp. of baking powder

Preparations:

1. Heat the oven to about 350°F and coat a muffin pan using paper liners.

2. Whisk the erythritol together with the almond flour, baking powder, cocoa powder, and salt inside a bowl dedicated to mixing.

3. Inside another bowl, whisk the eggs, cashew butter, and almond milk together.

4. Stir the wet Ingredients: to make them dry so that they become mixed, fold nuts in.

5. In a prepared pan, spoon the batter and place it in the oven for 22-25 minutes until a knife dipped in the middle comes out clean.

6. For the muffins in the pan, cool them for 5 minutes and then place them in a wire cooling rack.

Chocolate Protein Pancakes

Ingredients:

- 40g 2 scoop egg white protein powder
- Liquid stevia extract
- 1 teaspoon vanilla extract
- 1/2 cup unsweetened cocoa powder
- 1/2 cup coconut oil
- 1 cup canned coconut milk
- 8 large eggs

Preparations:

1. Mix the eggs, coconut oil, and coconut milk inside a food processor.
2. Beat the mixture for some period and then include the rest of the ingredients.
3. Blend the mixture so that it becomes very smooth and well mixed – set the sweetness to your choice.
4. Over medium heat, heat a nonstick skillet.

5. With about 1/2 cup for each pancake, spoon in the batter.

6. Heat and stop when bubbles form on the batter's surface, then mindfully flip.

7. Allow the pancake to cook so that the underside becomes colored brown.

8. Place in a plate to preserve it warm. Repeat with the rest of the batter.

Chive, Cheddar, Ham, And Omelet

Ingredients:

- 1 tbsp. of heavy cream
- 1/2 cup of shredded cheddar cheese
- Pepper and salt
- 1/2 cup of diced ham
- 3 whisked large eggs
- 1 tsp. of coconut oil
- 1 tbsp. of chopped chives

Preparations:

1. Whisk the chives, heavy cream, eggs, pepper, and salt together in a small bowl.
2. Heat the coconut oil inside a small skillet that is placed over medium heat.
3. Place the whisked eggs in and cook the mixture so that the bottom of the egg begins to set.

4. Tilt the pan to evenly distribute the eggs in the skillet and keep cooking until it becomes set.
5. Sprinkle the cheddar cheese and ham on half of the omelet and fold it over.
6. Allow the omelet to cook until the eggs are well set. Serve while hot.

Spinach Parmesan Egg Scramble

Ingredients:

- 1 tsp. of coconut oil

- 2 cups of fresh baby spinach

- 2 tbsp. of grated parmesan cheese

- 2 whisked large eggs

- 1 tbsp. of heavy cream

- Pepper and salt

Preparations:

1. Whisk the heavy cream together with the eggs, pepper, and salt inside a bowl.
2. Heat the coconut oil over medium heat, in a medium skillet.
3. Stir the spinach in and cook it for about 1 to 2 minutes until it is well wilted.
4. Pour the eggs in and cook it. Stir it occasionally, and keep cooking it for about 1 to 2 minutes until just set.

5. Stir the parmesan in and serve while it is hot.

Eggs And Russet Potatoes

Ingredients:

- Ginger 1 inch piece
- Olive oil 1 tablespoon
- Fresh Tomato sauce 15 oz.
- Cilantro
- Fresh Russet potatoes 2 lbs.
- Garlic 2 cloves
- Curry powder 2 tablespoons
- Eggs 4, large

Preparations:

1. Wash potatoes and then cut into cubes.
2. Heat water in a large pot and add potatoes; cook for 5 to 10 minutes or until tender.
3. Drain potatoes and put aside until needed cover to keep warm).
4. Prepare sauce by removing the peel from ginger and dice.

5. Heat oil in a deep, large skillet and add garlic and ginger; sauté for 2 minutes or until garlic is fragrant.
6. Put in curry and stir; cook for 1 minute.
7. Add tomato sauce and mix then lower heat and allow the sauce to cook until thoroughly heated.
8. Add potatoes to the mixture and use sauce to coat; add water if necessary.
9. Make 4 wells in potato mixture and break an egg into each.
10. Cover pot and cook for 5to 10 minutes or until eggs are set the way you prefer.
11. Serve topped with cilantro.

Turkey Chili

Ingredients:

- Ground turkey 1 lb., lean

- Bell pepper 1 red, chopped

- Fresh Tomato sauce 30 oz.

- Canned black beans 30 oz., drained and rinsed

- Jalapeno peppers 16 oz. jar, deli-sliced, drained

- Chili powder 2 tablespoons

- Olive oil 1 tablespoon

- Onion 1, chopped

- Bell pepper 1 yellow, chopped

- Canned tomatoes 30 oz., diced

- Canned kidney beans 30 oz., drained and rinsed

- Frozen corn 1 cup

- Cumin 1 tablespoon

Preparations:

1. Heat oil in a skillet and cook turkey until golden; transfer turkey to slow cooker.
2. Add peppers, tomatoes, jalapenos, cumin, onion, tomato sauce, beans, chili powder, and corn.
3. Set on low and cook for 4 to 6 hours or in high for 2 to 4 hours.
4. Serve as is or with desired toppings.

Almond Chicken Breast Saute

Ingredients:

- Broccoli florets 4 cups

- Green pepper 1, chopped

- Fresh Onion 2 cups, chopped

- Cherry tomatoes 2 cups, sliced in halves

- Pepper

- Chicken breasts 6 oz., sliced

- Olive oil 3 teaspoons

- Red pepper 1, chopped

- Garlic 2 cloves, diced

- Salt

- Almonds 4 teaspoons

Preparations:

1. Place broccoli in a steamer or pot and cook for 2 to 5 minutes; put aside until necessary.

2. Heat oil in a skillet and sauté peppers, garlic, chicken, and onion.
3. Cook for 10 to 15 minutes or until thoroughly cooked.
4. Add broccoli and tomatoes to chicken; stir to combine and add pepper and salt to taste.
5. Serve topped with almonds

Almond Cod Fish And Spinach

Ingredients:

- Lemon zest from 1 lemon

- Dill 1 tablespoon, fresh

- Pepper

- Dijon mustard 4 teaspoons

- Garlic 6 cloves, chopped

- Lemon juice freshly squeezed

- Onions 2 lbs.

- Vegetable stock 1 tablespoon, unsalted

- Balsamic vinegar 1/2 cup

- Almonds 1/2 cup, chopped

- Olive oil 2 teaspoons

- Codfish 1 lb.

- Water 1/4 cup

- Spinach 2 lbs.

- Olive oil 2 teaspoons

- Orange juice 1/2 cup, freshly squeezed

Preparations:

1. Heat a pot of water and add onions; leave in water for 10 to 15 seconds then drain and add cold water to onions and drain again.
2. Remove peels from onion and roots.
3. Heat stock and oil in a skillet and add onions; cook for 6 minutes until golden spots appear.
4. Put in vinegar and orange juice and heat until it boils.
5. Lower heat, stirring, and scraping bits from pot; cook for 5 to 10 minutes until tender use a knife to test onion).
6. Take onions from pot and put into a bowl and continue to boil for 1 to 2 minutes until mixture is syrupy.
7. Pour sauce on top of onion and cover to keep warm.
8. Set oven to 400°F and use cooking spray to coat a baking sheet.

9. Mix zest, dill, pepper, almonds, and 2 teaspoons of oil.

10. Use 1 teaspoon mustard to spread onto each piece of fish then press into the almond blend.

11. Bake for 5 to 10 minutes while heating stock in a pot.

12. Put in lemon juice, pepper and cook for 4 minutes.

13. Add garlic, stir and cook for 2 minutes.

14. Serve spinach along with fish.

Habanero And Bell Pepper Soup

Ingredients:

- Chicken broth 2 cups, low salt

- Tomatoes 2 lbs.

- Garlic 2 cloves, chopped

- Olive oil 1/4 cup, extra virgin

- Bell peppers 4 red, medium

- Sweet onion 1/2 lb., chopped

- Habanero peppers 6. Seeds removed and diced

Preparations:

1. Place bell peppers onto a greased baking sheet and broil for 10-15 minutes until blackened.
2. Take from heat and place into a bowl; cover the bowl with plastic wrap and put aside for 10 to 20 minutes.

3. Remove the peel and slice peppers in half; discard seeds and stems.

4. Use a knife to score tomatoes with an X on the bottom of each then heat a pot of water and place tomatoes into the pot for 10 to 20 seconds.

5. Take from hot water and place into an ice bath.

6. Remove peel and chop; put aside till needed.

7. Heat 2 tablespoons oil and sauté habaneros, garlic, and onion for 8 minutes or until golden and tender.

8. Put in bell peppers, tomatoes, and broth, cover, and cook for 5 minutes or until bell peppers are soft.

9. Add oil to soup and puree in 2 or more batches or use an immersion blender to puree in a pot then transfer soup to a metal bowl and chill in an ice bath, stirring frequently.

10. Serve.

Squash And Red Lentil

Ingredients:

- Ginger grated

- Sweet onion 1, chopped

- Curry powder 1 tablespoon

- Red lentils 1 cup

- Spinach 1 cup

- Herb seasoning 1/2 teaspoon

- Olive oil 1 teaspoon

- Garlic 3 cloves, diced

- Broth 4 cups, low salt

- Butternut squash 3 cups, cooked

Preparations:

1. Heat oil in a soup pot and sauté onion for 3 minutes or until soft.

2. Put in chilies, coriander, red peppers without liquid and cumin; cook for 2 minutes.

3. Add broth, liquid from peppers, and sweet potatoes.
4. Mix and bring to a boil, lower flame, and cover pot.
5. Cook for 10 to 15 minutes until potatoes are cooked.
6. Add lemon juice and cilantro; stir to combine and remove from heat.
7. Put cream cheese and half of the soup in a processor and blend smoothly then add the puree to remaining soup in pot and heat thoroughly,
8. Serve.

Chapter 5

Breakfast Recipes

Eggs And Sausage Breakfast Casserole

Ingredients:

- 2 cups milk

- 1/2 cup green onions, chopped

- Salt and pepper, to taste

- 1 pound bulk pork sausages, sliced

- 2 cups mozzarella cheese, shredded

- 8 fresh large eggs

Preparations:

1. Preheat the oven to 375ºF.

2. Cook the sausage in a pan for 6 minutes or until no longer pink.

3. Break them into crumbs and drain the oil.

4. Spread the sausage evenly in a cast-iron skillet and sprinkle cheese evenly.

5. Mix the milk and eggs in a bowl. Season with salt and pepper.

6. Pour the egg mixture over the sausage and cheese.

7. Bake in the oven for 30 to 35 minutes or until cooked.

8. Sprinkle with green onions and serve.

Sausage Quiche

Ingredients:

- 2 tbsp. fresh parsley, chopped

- 10 cherry tomatoes, halved

- 6 fresh eggs

- 2 tbsp. parmesan cheese, grated

- 5 eggplant slices

- 12 ounces pork sausage, chopped

- Salt and black pepper, to taste

- 2 tsp. whipping cream

Preparations:

1. Spread sausage pieces on a baking dish. Lay eggplant slices on top and add fresh cherry tomatoes.

2. In a bowl, mix eggs with salt, pepper, cream, and parmesan cheese. Whisk.

3. Pour into the baking dish. Place in the oven at 375ºF.

4. Bake for 35 to 40 minutes. Serve.

Mini Eggs In Cups

Ingredients:

- one cup cheddar cheese, shredded
- 1/2 cup green onion, chopped
- Cooking oil
- 6 eggs, beaten
- 1 tbsp. Dijon mustard
- two cup smoked salmon, finely chopped

Preparations:

1. Preheat the oven to 400ºF.
2. In a bowl, whisk the egg with the mustard. Set aside.
3. In another bowl, mix the smoked salmon, cheese, and green onions.
4. Grease a mini muffin pan with oil.
5. Place the egg mixture and salmon mixture into the muffin pan.

6. Bake for 10 to 20 minutes or until the eggs are set. Cool and serve.

Breakfast Skillet

Ingredients:

- 1 tbsp. coconut oil

- 1 tsp. garlic powder

- 1 tsp. dried basil

- 2 tbsp. Dijon mustard

- 2 zucchinis, chopped

- 8 ounces mushrooms, chopped

- Salt and black pepper, to taste

- 1 pound minced pork

Preparations:

1. Heat a pan with oil.
2. Add mushrooms and stir-fry for 2 to 4 minutes.
3. Add zucchini, salt, pepper, and stir-fry for 4 minutes.
4. Add pork, garlic powder, basil, salt, and pepper, and cook until meat is done.

5. Add mustard, stir, cook for 1 to 3 minutes.

6. Serve.

Blueberry Pancakes

Ingredients:

- 6 tbsp. coconut flour

- 2 tsp. baking powder

- 4 tbsp. cooking oil

- 1/2 cup blueberries

- 1 tsp. vanilla extract

- 2 eggs

Preparations:

1. In a bowl, mash the blueberries until only small bits remain.
2. Add the vanilla extract and eggs. Mix well.
3. Add the coconut flour and baking powder.
4. Add the cooking oil if the mixture is too dry.
5. Heat a pan and add a little oil.
6. Spoon 1/2 cup batter and lower the heat.
7. Cook 2 minutes per side.
8. Top with desired toppings and serve.

Chorizo And Cauliflower Breakfast

Ingredients:

- 1 cauliflower head, separated into florets

- 4 eggs, whisked

- 2 tbsp. green fresh onions, chopped

- 1 pound chorizo, chopped

- 12 ounces canned green chilies, chopped

- 1 onion, peeled and chopped

- 1 tsp. garlic powder

- Salt and black pepper, to taste

Preparations:

1. Heat a pan and add chorizo, onion.
2. Stir-fry until browned, about a few minutes.
3. Add green chilies. Stir-fry for a few minutes. Remove from heat.
4. In a food processor, mix cauliflower with some salt and pepper, and blend.

5. Transfer to a bowl, add eggs, salt, pepper, garlic powder, and chorizo mixture.

6. Whisk and transfer to a greased baking dish.

7. Bake in the oven at 375ºF for 35 to 40 minutes.

8. Cool and sprinkle green onions on top.

9. Slice and serve.

Bacon Avocado Breakfast Tacos

Ingredients:

- 3 Strips Bacon

- one Avocado

- 1 Oz. Cheddar Cheese, Shredded

- Salt And Pepper

- 1 C. Mozzarella Cheese, Shredded

- six fresh Eggs

- 2 Tbsp. Butter

Preparations:

1. Preheat the oven to 375 degrees and cook the bacon on a baking sheet for twenty minutes.

2. As the bacon cooks, heat a third of a cup of the cheese at a time in a pan on medium heat to make the shells.

3. When the cheese is brown on the edges, use some tongs to lift it and drape it over a wooden spoon over the opening of a pot.

4. Do the same with the rest of the cheese to make three shells.
5. Cook the eggs in the butter and stir until they're done. Season to taste.
6. Spoon a third of the eggs, bacon, and avocado into the hardened shells.
7. Sprinkle the cheddar over the tops and add a little cilantro and hot sauce.

Chive, Bacon, And Cheddar Omelet

Ingredients:

- 1 Oz. Cheddar Cheese
- two Chive Stalks
- Salt And Pepper
- 2 Bacon Slices, Cooked
- one Tsp. Bacon Fat
- 2 fresh Eggs

Preparations:

1. Be sure everything is prepared and then heat a pan over medium-low with the bacon fat.
2. Add the eggs and season with salt and pepper and the chives.
3. Once the edges begin to set, add the bacon to the center and cook for thirty seconds. Turn the stove off.

4. Add the cheese on the bacon and fold the edges in toward the center, holding them in place until the cheese melts.

5. Flip and warm on the other side.

Egg Cups

Ingredients:

- 4 Jalapenos, Chopped
- 1 Tsp. Onion Powder
- 1 Tsp. Garlic Powder
- Salt And Pepper
- 12 Bacon Strips
- 8 Eggs
- 4 Oz. Cheddar Cheese
- 3 Oz. Cream Cheese

Preparations:

1. Preheat your oven to 375 degrees and par-cook the bacon so it's crisp but still pliable.
2. Save the grease to add it to the cup mix.
3. Use a mixer to mix everything else, except the cheese and a jalapeno.
4. Grease the muffin tin and put the bacon around the edges.

5. Pour the egg mix into the wells and add the cheese and a jalapeno ring to each cup.

6. Cook at 375 degrees for twenty-five minutes.

7. Once it's cooked, remove it from the oven and allow it to cool.

Cinnamon Roll Oatmeal

Ingredients:

- 3 Tbsp. Butter
- 1 Tsp. Maple Flavor
- 2 Tsp. Cinnamon
- 1/2 Tsp. Nutmeg
- 1 Tsp. Vanilla
- 1/2 Tsp. Allspice
- 1 C. Crushed Pecans
- 1 C. Flax Seed
- 1 C. Chia Seed
- 1 C. Cauliflower, Riced
- 4 C. Coconut Milk
- 1/2 C. Heavy Cream
- 3 Oz. Cream Cheese

Preparations:

1. Rice the cauliflower in a food processor and then set it aside.
2. Begin heating the milk in a pan over medium heat.
3. Crush the pecans and toast them in the pan.
4. Add the coconut milk and cauliflower together and bring them to a boil.
5. Add the spices and mix them.
6. Add the flax and chia seeds and mix this.
7. Add the butter, cream, cream cheese, and mix it again.

Chive, Cheddar, And Ham Soufflé

Ingredients:

- 6 fresh Eggs

- 1 C. Cheddar Cheese, Shredded

- 1 C. Heavy Cream

- 3 Tbsp. Fresh Chives, Chopped

- 1 Tsp. Kosher Salt

- 1/2 Tsp. Black Pepper

- 3 Tbsp. Olive Oil

- 1 fresh Onion, Diced

- 2 Tsp. Garlic, Minced

- 6 Oz. Ham Steak, Cubed And Cooked

- 1 Tbsp. Butter

Preparations:

1. Preheat your oven to 400 degrees and heat the oil in the pan.

2. Add the onions, and once they're soft, add the garlic. Brown them.
3. In a bowl, add the other Ingredients: and mix them well.
4. Separate the mix into the greased ramekins and bake them for twenty minutes.
5. Let them cool and serve.

Spinach Omelet

Ingredients:

- 2 Tbsp. Heavy Cream
- 1 Oz. Goat Cheese
- 1 Spring Onion
- Salt And Pepper
- 1/2 fresh Onion
- 2 Tbsp. Butter
- 1 C. Spinach
- 3 fresh Eggs

Preparations:

1. Slice the onion into strips. Sauté it in the butter until it's caramelized and add the spinach to the pan. Let it wilt.
2. Remove the vegetables and mix the three eggs, cream, salt, and pepper into a container and mix.

3. Pour the egg mix into the pan and let it cook over medium heat.
4. When the edges start to set, spoon the onion and spinach over half the omelet.
5. Crumble the cheese over the spinach and as the top begins to set, fold it and serve.
6. Garnish with the spring onions.

Cheese And Sausage Breakfast Pie

Ingredients:

- 5 Egg Yolks

- 2 Tsp. Lemon Juice

- 1/2 Tsp. Cayenne Pepper

- 1 Tsp. Rosemary

- 1 Tsp. Kosher Salt

- 1/2 Tsp. Baking Soda

- 2 Sausage Cheddar And Bacon Flavored)

- 2 C. Cheddar Cheese, Grated

- 1/2 C. Coconut Flour

- 1/2 C. Coconut Oil

- 2 Tbsp. Coconut Milk

Preparations:

1. Cube the sausage and fry it over medium heat. Preheat your oven to 350 degrees in the meantime.

2. Separate the egg yolks and discard the whites.

3. Measure out the dry spices and flour into a bowl.

4. Mix everything until it's combined.

5. Beat the yolks until they're creamy, around four to five minutes. Add the milk, oil, and lemon juice and keep beating.

6. Add the wet to the dry and fold half a cup of the cheese into the batter.

7. Measure the batter into two ramekins and fill them about three-quarters of the way full.

8. When the sausage is done, poke the sausage into the batter and make sure it's evenly distributed.

9. Bake for twenty-five minutes or until the tops are browned.

10. Sprinkle the rest of the cheese on top and broil for four minutes.

Egg Baskets

Ingredients:

- 6 Tbsp. Salsa

- 1 Tsp. Paprika

- 1 Tsp. Pepper

- 1 Tsp. Salt

- 1/2 Tsp. Cayenne Pepper

- 2 C. Cheese

- 6 Bacon Slices

- 3 Tbsp. Bacon Fat

- 6 Eggs

Preparations:

1. Place a quarter of a cup of cheese onto a silicone baking tray and put them in the oven at 400 degrees for ten minutes.

2. When they come out, mold them into a cup or keep them flat.

3. In the pan, crisp your bacon.

4. Once it's crisp, remove it to some paper towels and leave the grease in the pan.

5. Fry some eggs in the pan.

6. Use a metal ramekin to remove any excess egg white to make a circular pattern or leave the egg misshapen.

7. Put the fried egg on the cheese crisp and top with a tablespoon of salsa and some extra bacon.

8. Scramble three eggs in the rest of the fat and make some scrambled egg cups and top with a tablespoon of salsa and some extra bacon.

Chapter 6

Keto Salad Recipes

Mixed Green Spring Salad

Ingredients:

- 2 Tbsp. Raspberry Vinaigrette

- 2 Bacon Slices

- Salt And Pepper

- 2 Oz. Mixed Greens

- 3 Tbsp. Pine Nuts, Roasted

- 2 Tbsp. Shaved Parmesan

Preparations:

1. Cook the bacon until it's crisp.

2. Crumble and add it to the salad with the remaining ingredients.

3. Shake the dressing and place it over the salad. Serve.

Pork Salad

Ingredients:

- 2 Tbsp. Cilantro, Chopped

- 1 Tsp. Red Curry Paste

- 1 Tsp. Five Spice

- 1 Tbsp. Rice Wine Vinegar

- 1 Tsp. Fish Sauce

- 1/2 Tsp. Red Pepper Flakes

- 1 Tsp. Mango Extract

- 10 Oz. Pulled Pork

- 2 C. Romaine Lettuce

- 1/2 C. Cilantro, Chopped

- 1/2 Red Bell Pepper, Chopped

- 2 Tbsp. Tomato Paste

- 1 Tbsp. Creamy Peanut Butter

- 2 Tbsp. Soy Sauce

- Juice & Zest Of 1 Lime

Preparations:

1. Zest the lime and chop the cilantro. In a bowl, combine the tomato paste through the mango extract together.
2. Use your finger to pull apart the pork.
3. Assemble the salad and glaze it with the sauce.

Caprese Salad

Ingredients:

- 3 Tbsp. Olive Oil

- Black Pepper

- Salt

- 1 fresh Tomato

- 6 Oz. Fresh Mozzarella Cheese

- 1/2 C. Fresh Basil, Chopped

Preparations:

1. Chop the basil with the olive oil in a food processor to make a paste.
2. Slice the tomato.
3. Cut the mozzarella into one-ounce slices.
4. Assemble the salad by putting down one slice of fresh tomato, a slice of cheese, and then top with the basil.
5. Season to taste and enjoy.

Cucumber Salad

Ingredients:

- 1 Tbsp. Sesame Oil

- 1/2 Tsp. Red Pepper Flakes

- 1 Tsp. Sesame Seeds

- 1 Tbsp. Rice Vinegar

- Salt And Pepper

- two Cucumber

- 1 Packet Shirataki Noodles

- two Tbsp. Coconut Oil

- 1 Spring Onion

Preparations:

1. Rinse the noodles well. Be sure you get any excess water off.

2. Set them on a paper towel and let them dry.

3. Add two tablespoons of coconut oil to a pan and bring to medium heat.

4. Once the pan's hot, fry the noodles for seven minutes.

5. Remove from the pan and put them on a paper towel to drain.

6. Slice the cucumbers and arrange them on a plate.

7. Add the remaining ingredient and let it rest half an hour in the refrigerator.

8. Sprinkle the noodles over the top and serve.

Spinach Salad

Ingredients:

- three Tbsp. Parmesan Cheese
- 1 Tsp. Red Pepper Flakes
- six C. Spinach
- 1/2 C. Ranch Dressing

Preparations:

1. Add the spinach to a bowl and drench with the ranch dressing.
2. Mix it and add the red pepper flakes and the parmesan.
3. Mix it again and serve.

Egg Salad

Ingredients:

- 1/2 Red Onion

- 2 Tsp. Dijon Mustard

- 1/2 Tsp. Black Pepper

- 1/2 Tsp. Cayenne Pepper

- 5 Eggs, Hard Boiled

- 1/2 C. Mayonnaise

- three Bacon Slices

- 2 Tbsp. Bacon Fat

Preparations:

1. Slice the bacon into thin slices and cook them over medium heat in a pan until they're crispy.
2. As the bacon cooks, slice the red onion.
3. Take out the bacon and leave the drippings behind.
4. Drain the bacon on paper towels.

5. Add the bacon drippings, a quarter of a cup of mayonnaise, two tablespoons of the mustard, and the red onion to the eggs.

6. Mix it well and smash the eggs.

7. Add the spices. Add the bacon.

8. Fold and mix. Serve and enjoy.

Chapter 7

Keto Main Dish Recipes

Mandarin Chicken W/ Homemade Orange Sauce

Ingredients:

Chicken:

- 1 tablespoon Chinese 5-Spice

- Pinch of salt

- 6 chicken thighs

Orange sauce:

- 1 cup sugar-free orange marmalade

- 2 tablespoons Red Boat fish sauce

- 1 tablespoon fresh minced ginger

- 1 tablespoon fresh orange juice

- 1 tablespoon granulated stevia

- 1 teaspoon coconut aminos

- 1 teaspoon ground garlic

- 1 teaspoon red pepper flakes

Preparations:

1. Season thighs with 5-spice and salt.

2. Heat a skillet.

3. When very hot, add thighs, skin-side down first, and brown for 1 to 3 minutes on each side. Add to slow cooker.

4. Mix all the sauce Ingredients: in a bowl and pour over chicken.

5. Close the lid.

6. Cook on low for 6 hours.

Ginger + Coconut-Spiced Chicken

Ingredients:

- 2-inch piece of ginger, grated

- Salt and pepper to taste

- 2 cup full-fat coconut milk

- 4 minced garlic cloves

Preparation:

1. Pour coconut milk, garlic, and ginger into your slow cooker.

2. Season chicken with salt and pepper.

3. Put chicken in the slow cooker, spooning over the milk mixture.

4. Close the lid.

5. Cook on low for 6-8 hours.

6. When Times up, remove the chicken and pull the meat off the bones.

7. Put meat back in the slow cooker and heat through.

8. Add more seasonings if needed.

9. Serve!

Turkey Gravy

Ingredients:

- 1 tablespoon olive oil

- 1 tablespoon Italian seasoning

- 2 teaspoons arrowroot powder

- Salt to taste

- two cups chicken stock

- Four chopped celery stalks

- 3 chopped carrots

- one big chopped onion

Preparations:

1. Season turkey well with Italian seasoning.
2. Heat olive oil in a skillet until very hot, and then sear turkey for 2 to 5 minutes on each side.
3. Put turkey in your slow cooker.
4. Pour the stock into the skillet and deglaze, scraping up any meat bits.

5. Pour into the slow cooker.

6. Add onions, celery, and carrots.

7. Close the lid.

8. Cook on low for 5-6 hours, until turkey has cooked evenly to 165-degrees.

9. Now, it is time to make the gravy.

10. Remove the turkey breast and veggies, tenting with foil on a plate.

11. Pour cooking liquid through a strainer into a saucepan.

12. Turn the burner on and heat until boiling, then reduce.

13. Mix 1-2 tablespoons of cold water with the arrowroot powder.

14. When the liquid is just simmering, stir slowly into the saucepan.

15. It should begin to thicken. Once thick, remove from the heat.

16. Taste and add salt if needed.

17. Serve turkey and veggies with gravy!

Cheesy Turkey "Pasta"

Ingredients:

- 1 teaspoon cumin

- 1 teaspoon dried parsley

- Salt and pepper to taste

- A sprinkle of parmesan cheese

- 1 pound cooked and shredded turkey breast

- 1 cup mozzarella cheese

- 3 minced garlic cloves

- 1 diced onion

Sauce:

- 1 tablespoon grass-fed butter

- 1 cup mozzarella cheese

- 2 cup heavy cream

Preparations:

1. Mix spaghetti squash, turkey, onion, garlic, and seasonings into your slow cooker.

84

2. Put butter in a skillet, and melt.

3. Whisk in cream, gradually pouring it in.

4. Add cheese, still stirring, until melted.

5. Pour into the slow cooker and mix.

6. Cook on high for 2-3 hours.

7. Garnish with a sprinkle of Parmesan cheese and serve!

Turkey-Stuffed Bell Peppers

Ingredients:

- 1 cup water

- 2 teaspoons Italian seasoning

- Salt and pepper to taste

- 1 pound ground turkey

- 3 cups low carb tomato sauce like Rao"s)

- 1 minced onion

- 2 minced garlic cloves

Preparations:

1. Begin by cleaning the peppers and cutting off the tops.
2. In a bowl, mix two tablespoons of sauce, onion, garlic, Italian seasoning, and turkey.
3. Stuff meat mixture into peppers.
4. Put filled peppers in your slow cooker.
5. Pour in 1 cup of water around peppers.
6. Spoon remaining sauce on top of peppers.

7. Close the lid. Cook on low for 6-8 hours.

8. When Time up, taste, and season with salt and pepper if needed.

9. Serve!

Beef Bourguignon

Ingredients:

- 2 bay leaves

- 1 tablespoon tomato paste no sugar added)

- 1 teaspoon dried parsley

- 1 teaspoon dried thyme

- Salt and pepper to taste

- One 750ml bottle of dry red wine

- 4 cups sliced mushrooms

- 8 slices bacon

- One diced onion

- 3 tablespoons grass-fed butter

- three minced garlic cloves

Preparations:

1. If the beef is "t cut yet, chop it into chunks.

2. Season well with salt and pepper.

3. Heat 2 tablespoons of butter in a skillet.

4. When hot, add beef and cook for 3 minutes on each side.

5. Remove beef and put it into a slow cooker.

6. Add bacon and cook until crisp. Remove bacon and chop.

7. Pour a bit of red wine into the skillet to deglaze by scraping up any stuck-on meat.

8. Put bacon in your slow cooker, and pour in the contents of the skillet and the rest of the wine.

9. Add all the other Ingredients: and stir.

10. Cook on low for 8-10 hours, until meat is tender.

11. Serve hot!

Easiest Short Ribs

Ingredients:

- 2 minced garlic cloves

- 1 bay leaf

- Salt and pepper to taste

- eight tablespoons grass-fed butter

- 1 cup beef stock

Preparations:

1. Trim the ribs so each piece has just one bone in it.

2. Put everything in your slow cooker.

3. Close the lid.

4. Cook on low for 5-6 hours. Serve!

Slow-Cooker Swiss Steak Veggies

Ingredients:

- 1 cup sliced onions

- three minced garlic cloves

- Salt and pepper to taste

- One 14.5-ounce can of diced tomatoes

- 2 cups beef stock

- 1 cup sliced mushrooms

- 1 cup sliced carrots

Preparations:

1. Just put everything in your slow cooker and stir.
2. Close the lid. Cook on low for 8-1o hours.
3. Enjoy!

Cider-Braised Beef Shank

Ingredients:

- 5 minced garlic cloves

- 1 bay leaf

- 1 tablespoon extra virgin olive oil

- Salt and pepper to taste

- four cups beef stock

- three cups apple cider

- 2 chopped onions

Preparations:

1. Dry your beef shanks and season well with salt and pepper.
2. Add oil to a skillet and heat.
3. When hot, brown the shank for 5 to 7 minutes per side.
4. Put meat in the slow cooker.
5. Add garlic and onion to the skillet and cook until fragrant.

6. Pour in the stock and deglaze by scraping up any stuck-on food.

7. Pour into the slow cooker with cider.

8. Add the rest of the Ingredients.

9. Close the lid. Cook on low for 6-8 hours.

10. Serve when meat is tender.

Coconut-Ginger Beef

Ingredients:

- 2 minced garlic cloves
- 1 teaspoon ground ginger
- Salt and pepper to taste
- two cup full-fat coconut milk
- 1 tablespoon red curry paste

Preparations:

1. In a bowl, mix coconut milk, curry paste, garlic, ginger, and salt and pepper.
2. Pour into slow cooker.
3. Add beef and turn over in the mixture to coat.
4. Close the lid. Cook on low for 6-7 hours.
5. Taste and season more if necessary before serving.

Classic Pot Roast

Ingredients:

- 3 minced garlic cloves

- 1 cup red wine

- 1 tablespoon extra virgin olive oil

- Salt and pepper to taste

- 1 chopped onion

- 4 sliced celery stalks

- 3 big sliced carrots

Preparations:

1. Pat your beef dry.

2. Season well with salt and pepper.

3. Heat oil in a pan and add meat to sear, about 2 to 5 minutes per side or until golden.

4. Put all the Ingredients: in your slow cooker, including meat. Close the lid.

5. Cook on low for 8 hours.

6. When Time up, shred the meat and then cook for another half hour. Serve!

Italian-Style Pot Roast

Ingredients:

- one tablespoon no-sugar tomato paste

- 3 minced garlic cloves

- 1 tablespoon salt-free Italian seasoning

- 1 teaspoon ground nutmeg

- Salt and pepper to taste

- two cups beef stock

- two cups chopped carrots

- 1 chopped onion

- 2 cups crushed tomatoes

Preparations:

1. If your beef is "t cubed yet, chop.
2. Put into your pot.
3. Add onions, carrots, garlic, and seasonings.
4. Add tomatoes, paste, and stock. Stir well.
   Close the lid.

5. Cook on low for 8 hours. When meat is tender, serve!

Cinnamon Roll Waffles

Ingredients:

- 1 tsp. of ground cinnamon

- 1 tsp. of vanilla extract

- 1 cup of heavy cream

- A pinch of ground nutmeg

- 3 tbsp. of coconut flour

- 4 large fresh eggs, divided into yolks and whites

- 3 tbsp. of powdered erythritol

- two tsp. of baking powder

Preparations:

1. Separate the eggs into two different mixing bowls.
2. Whip the egg whites until stiff peaks form then set aside.

3. Whisk the egg yolks with coconut flour, erythritol, baking powder, vanilla, cinnamon, and nutmeg in the other bowl.

4. Add the heavy cream, whisking until just combined, then gently fold in the egg whites.

5. Preheat the waffle iron and grease with cooking spray.

6. Spoon about 1 cup of batter into the iron.

7. Cook the waffle according to the manufacturer's instructions.

8. Remove the waffle to a plate and repeat with the remaining batter.

Bacon Swiss Waffles

Ingredients:

- 3 tbsp. of unsweetened almond milk

- Pepper and salt

- 1/2 cup of sour cream

- 1 cup of shredded Swiss cheese

- 4 large eggs, divided into yolks and whites

- six slices of uncooked bacon

- three tbsp. of coconut flour

- 2 tsp. of baking powder

Preparations:

1. Put the bacon inside a skillet and heat it so that it becomes crispy.
2. Coarsely chop it in a bowl.
3. Measure about 3 tbsp. of the bacon grease and reserve it.
4. Divide the eggs into two separate mixing bowls.

5. Beat in the egg whites until it starts to form stiff peaks. Set it aside.

6. Whisk in the egg yolks with the baking powder, erythritol, coconut flour, pepper, and salt in the other bowl.

7. Add the bacon grease and almond milk to the second bowl while whisking.

8. Gently fold the egg whites in and stop when it is just combined.

9. Stir in half of the chopped bacon and the shredded Swiss cheese.

10. Heat the grease and waffle iron making use of the cooking spray.

11. Spoon out a half cup of batter into the iron.

12. After reading the manufacturer's instructions, cook the waffle accordingly.

13. Place the waffle on a plate and replicate with the rest of the batter.

14. Top the waffles with chopped bacon and sour cream. Serve.

Spinach Cauliflower Soup

Ingredients:

- three cups of vegetable broth
- 8 oz. of chopped fresh baby spinach
- Pepper and salt
- 1 cup of canned coconut milk
- 1 chopped small yellow onion
- 1 tbsp. of coconut oil
- 2 cups of chopped cauliflower
- 2 cloves of minced garlic

Preparations:

1. Over medium-high heat, heat the coconut oil in a saucepan– include the garlic and fresh onion.
2. Stir in the cauliflower after Sautéing for 4-5 minutes till it turns brown.

3. Place over heat and cook for about 2 to 5 minutes, stir in the baby spinach when it turns brown.

4. Allow it to cook for another 2 minutes until it becomes wilted.

5. Stir in the broth and allow it to boil.

6. Take out from the heat and use an immersion blender to puree the soup.

7. Stir the coconut milk in and garnish with pepper and salt to taste. Serve.

Cheesy Buffalo Chicken Sandwich

Ingredients:

- 1 oz. of softened cream cheese

- 1 cup of cooked and shredded chicken breast

- 2 tbsp. of hot sauce

- 1 slice Swiss cheese

- 1 fresh large egg, separated into white and yolk

- Pinch cream of tartar

- Pinch salt

Preparations:

1. Heat the oven to about 300°F for the bread and coat the baking sheet using parchment paper.

2. Whip in the cream of tartar with the egg whites and add salt till soft peaks start to form.

3. Whisk the egg yolk and cream cheese until it is pale yellow and smooth.

4. Carefully fold in the egg whites until it is well combined and smooth.

5. Spoon the batter into two equal circles on the top of the baking sheet.

6. Place in the oven and bake for 20 to 25 minutes until lightly browned and firm.

7. Shred the chicken into a toss and bowl with the hot sauce.

8. Spoon the chicken on the top of one of the bread circles and garnish it with cheese.

9. Top it with the extra bread circle. Serve and enjoy.

Coconut Chicken Tenders

Ingredients:

- 1 teaspoon garlic powder

- 2 pounds boneless chicken tenders

- Salt and pepper

- 2 fresh large eggs, whisked well

- 1/2 cup almond flour

- 2 tablespoons shredded unsweetened coconut

Preparations:

1. Heat the oven to about 400°F and coat a baking sheet using parchment.

2. Stir the garlic powder, coconut, and almond flour inside a shallow dish together.

3. Season the chicken with pepper and salt, then place the chicken into the whipped eggs.

4. Dredge the chicken tenders inside the mixture of almond flour, set it on the baking sheet.

5. Bake it for about 25-30 minutes until it cooks through and appears brown. Serve hot.

Avocado Spinach Salad With Almonds

Ingredients:

- 2 tsp. of balsamic vinegar

- 1 thinly sliced medium avocado

- Pepper and salt

- 1/2 cup of sliced and toasted almonds

- 2 tsp. of olive oil

- four cups of fresh baby spinach

- 1 tsp. of Dijon mustard

Preparations:

1. Toss the baby spinach with the Dijon mustard, balsamic vinegar, olive oil, pepper and salt.

2. Share the spinach in between two plates of salad.

3. Top the salads using toasted almonds and sliced avocado. Serve.

Easy Chopped Salad

Ingredients:

- 1 cup of halved cherry tomatoes
- 1 cup of shredded cheddar cheese
- 2 sliced and peeled hardboiled eggs
- 1 cup of diced ham
- 1 small chopped and pitted avocado
- four cups of fresh lettuce that is chopped
- 1/2 cup of diced cucumber

Preparations:

1. Share the lettuce among the two salad bowls or plates.
2. Top the salads with diced celery, tomato, and. avocado
3. Include the shredded cheese, diced ham, and sliced egg.
4. Serve the salads using your preferred keto-friendly dressing.

Cauliflower Leek Soup With Pancetta

Ingredients:

- 1.2 cup of sliced leeks

- 2 oz. of diced pancetta

- Salt and pepper

- 1 chopped medium head cauliflower

- 4 cups of chicken broth

- 1 cup of heavy cream

Preparations:

1. Mix the cauliflower and broth inside a saucepan that is placed over medium-high heat.

2. Heat the chicken broth until it begins to boil. Add the sliced leeks.

3. Keep it covered and allow it to keep boiling for 1 hour till when the cauliflower becomes tender.

4. Take out from heat and use an immersion blender to puree the soup.

5. Stir the cream in, then season with pepper and salt.

6. In a skillet placed over medium-high heat, fry the pancetta that was chopped until it becomes crispy.

7. Place the soup into the bowls and garnish with pancetta. Serve.

Three Meat And Cheese Sandwich

Ingredients:

- 1 oz. of sliced hard salami
- 1 oz. of sliced ham
- 2 slices of cheddar cheese
- 1 oz. of sliced turkey
- Pinch cream of tartar
- 1 large egg, separated
- 1 oz. of softened cream cheese
- Pinch salt

Preparations:

1. For the bread Preparations, heat the oven to about 300°F and coat a baking sheet using parchment.
2. Whip the cream of tartar with the egg whites and salt and stop when soft peaks form.
3. Whisk in the egg yolk and cream cheese until it becomes pale yellow and smooth.

4. Carefully fold the egg white in, one at a time, until it becomes well combined and smooth.

5. Spoon the batter on the baking sheet into two equal circles.

6. Place in the oven and bake for about 20 to 25 minutes until it is lightly browned and firm.

7. Layer the cheeses and sliced meats in between the bread circles to finish the sandwich.

8. Lubricate a skillet using cooking spray and place it over medium heat.

9. Include the sandwich and cook until underneath appears browned, then turn and cook and stop when the cheese just melts.

Chicken Caesar Salad Wrap

Ingredients:

- Flatbread/Tortillas 2

- Curly kale 6 cups, chopped

- Vegan Parmesan 3/4 cup, shredded

- Garlic 1 clove, diced

- Honey 1 teaspoon

- Olive oil 1/8 cup

- Grilled chicken 8 oz., sliced thin

- Cherry tomatoes 1 cup, cut into quarters

- Coddled egg 1/2

- Dijon mustard 1/2 teaspoon

- Lemon juice 1/8 cup, freshly squeezed

Preparations:

1. Put coddled egg, mustard, lemon juice, olive oil, and garlic together in a bowl; whisk together until thoroughly combined.

2. Add tomatoes, chicken, and kale to mixture and coat then add 1/2 cup of cheese.
3. Divide salad in 2 and spoon onto tortillas/flatbread and top with 1/4cup cheese each.
4. Roll wraps and cuts in half.
5. Serve.

Spiced Carrot Ginger Soup

Ingredients:

- Mustard seeds 1/2 teaspoon, yellow

- Curry powder 1/2 teaspoon

- Onion 2 cups, chopped

- Lime zest 2 teaspoons

- Lime juice 2 teaspoons, freshly squeezed

- Coriander seeds 1 teaspoon

- Peanut oil 3 tablespoons

- Ginger 1 tablespoon, peeled and diced

- Carrots 2 lbs., sliced thin into rounds

- Chicken broth 6 cups, low salt

Preparations:

1. Grind mustard seeds and coriander together finely.

2. Heat oil in a large soup pot and add curry powder along with ground mixture then add ginger and cook for 1 minute.

3. Add zest, fresh onion, and carrots; cook for 3 minutes until onions are soft then add broth and heat until mixture boils.

4. Lower heat and cook for 25 to 30 minutes until carrots are cooked. Remove from heat and allow to cool.

5. Puree in batches or use an immersion blender to puree.

6. Reheat, adding more liquid if necessary along with lime juice.

7. Serve.

Seared Salmon With Baby Arugula

Ingredients:

- Salmon 2 center-cut filets

- Olive oil 2 tablespoons

- Black pepper

- Fresh Lemon juice 2 tablespoons

- All-purpose seasoning 1/8 teaspoon

For salad:

- Baby arugula 3 cups

- Red onion 1/4 cup, sliced

- Olive oil 1 tablespoon, extra virgin

- Cherry tomatoes 2/3 cup, cut in half

- Black pepper

- Wine vinegar 1 tablespoon

Preparations:

1. Season fish with all-purpose, oil and lemon juice; marinate for 10 to 15 minutes.
2. Heat skillet and place the salmon onto the skin side into the pot and cook for 3 minutes. Use a spatula to lightly lift fish to avoid sticking.
3. Lower heat and cover pan; cook for 2 to 4 minutes until skin is crispy.
4. Combine fresh onion, tomatoes, and arugula in a bowl then drizzle with vinegar and oil.
5. Serve salad with fish.

Goat Cheese And Bell Pepper Salad

Ingredients:

- Fresh Lemon juice 2 tablespoons, freshly squeezed

- Spinach leaves 4 cups, chopped

- Red onion 1/3 cup, chopped

- Celery 2 cups, chopped

- Olive oil 2 tablespoons, extra-virgin

- Oregano 1 tablespoon, chopped

- Red peppers 2 large, diced

- Goat cheese 3/4 cup, soft, crumbled

Preparations:

1. Put oregano, lemon juice, and oil in a bowl and whisk together.
2. Add remaining ingredients: to dressing and toss.
3. Serve. May be chilled before serving.

Fusil Salad

Ingredients:

- Olive oil 1 teaspoon, extra-virgin

- Fresh Onion 1/2, chopped

- Bell pepper 1/2, chopped

- Canned tomatoes 7 oz., diced

- Basil 1/4 teaspoon, chopped

- Lemon juice 1 tablespoon, freshly squeezed

- Fusil 3/4 cups, organic

- Celery 1/2 stalk, chopped

- Garlic 1 clove, diced

- Ground turkey 1.5 oz., lean

- Red pepper flakes 1/4 teaspoon

- Black pepper

- Water 1 tablespoon

For Salad:

- Olive oil 1/2 teaspoon

- Bell pepper 1/4, sliced

- Lettuce 1/2 cup

- Cucumber 1/4 cup

Preparations:

1. Cook fusil for 2 to 4 minutes, drain and put aside.

2. Heat oil in a skillet and sauté onion and celery for 3 minutes then add bell pepper and garlic; take from the pot and put aside.

3. Use cooking spray to coat the pot and cook turkey for 2 to 5 minutes or until thoroughly golden.

4. Add fusil and cooked vegetables to the pot along with crushed pepper and canned tomatoes; mix, cover, and cook for 3 to 8 minutes.

5. Top with basil and serve.

6. Combine Ingredients: for salad and serve alongside chop sue.

Cream Cheese Chive Omelet

Ingredients:

- 1 tbsp. olive oil

- Salt and pepper, to taste

- Water, as needed

- 4 fresh large eggs

- 2 tbsp. minced chives

- 2 ounces cream cheese, cubed

Preparations:

1. Heat the oil in a skillet.
2. In a bowl, whisk the eggs, chives, salt, and pepper.
3. Add water if necessary.
4. Add the egg mixture into the skillet.
5. Cook until set. Tilt the skillet so the egg cooks well.
6. Then sprinkle cheese on one side and fold the eggs. Slice and serve.

Spanish Omelet

Ingredients:

- 2 tbsp. cilantro, chopped
- 1 tbsp. oil
- Salsa for garnish
- 6 fresh large eggs
- 1/2 cup red onion, chopped
- 1 cup Mexican cheese blend, divided

Preparations:

1. Heat oil in a skillet
2. Whisk the eggs in a bowl. Add the egg mixture into the skillet. Allow it to set.
3. When the eggs are set, spoon the fresh onion on one side.
4. Sprinkle with cheese. Fold the eggs and allow them to cook.
5. Garnish and serve.

Spinach And Mushroom Omelet

Ingredients:

- 1 cup baby spinach, chopped

- 2 tbsp. provolone cheese, shredded

- Salt and pepper, to taste

- 4 large eggs

- 1 tsp. butter

- 1 cup thinly sliced fresh mushrooms, chopped

Preparations:

1. Beat the eggs. Season with salt and pepper. Set aside.
2. Heat butter in a skillet. Sauté the mushrooms for 3 minutes.
3. Add the spinach and cook until wilted.
4. Stir in the eggs and the cheese.
5. Cook until done. Serve.

Keto Bacon And Egg Casserole

Ingredients:

- 12 large eggs, beaten
- Salt and pepper, to taste
- 12 bacon strips, diced
- 1/2 cup fresh butter

Preparations:

1. Cook the bacon on a skillet until the fat has been rendered.
2. Take the bacon out and place it on paper towels to drain excess fat.
3. Heat butter until melted.
4. Pour in the egg and season with salt and pepper.
5. Stir in the bacon.
6. Cover with foil and bake in the oven at 400ºF for 10 to 20 minutes or until the eggs have set.

7. Serve.

Mexican Breakfast

Ingredients:

- 1 pound ground pork

- 1 pound chorizo, chopped

- Salt and black pepper, to taste

- 8 eggs

- 1 fresh tomato, cored and chopped

- 3 tbsp. butter

- 1 cup fresh onion, chopped

- 1 avocado, chopped

- 1 cup fresh tomato paste

- 1 tsp. garlic powder

- 1 tsp. dried basil

- 1 tsp. dried oregano

- 1 tsp. cumin

- 2 tsp. chili powder

Preparations:

1. In a bowl, mix tomato paste and spices to make enchilada sauce.
2. In another bowl, mix chorizo and pork.
3. Stir and spread on a lined baking sheet.
4. Spread enchilada sauce on top, place in the oven at 350ºF, and bake for 10 to 20 minutes.
5. Heat a pan with butter and add eggs, and scramble them.
6. Take pork mixture out of the oven and spread scrambled eggs over them.
7. Sprinkle fresh onion, tomato, salt, pepper, and avocado on top.
8. Serve.

Keto Smoothie

Ingredients:

- 1 tsp. chia seeds

- 2 tsp. unsweetened cocoa powder

- 1 tsp almond butter

- 2 cups Thai coconut milk

- 1 tsp. low-carb sweetener

- 1/2 avocado, chopped

- 1 cup blackberries

Preparations:

1. Place all Ingredients: in a blender.
2. Blend until smooth.

Coconut Porridge

Ingredients:

- 1 pinch nutmeg

- 1 cup almonds, ground

- 1 tbsp. coconut flour

- 1 tsp. stevia

- 2 cup coconut cream

- A pinch of ground cardamom

- A pinch of ground cloves

- 1 tsp. ground cinnamon

Preparations:

1. Heat a pan over medium heat.
2. Add coconut cream and heat for a few minutes.
3. Add coconut flour, almonds, and stevia. Mix well and cook for 2 to 5 minutes.
4. Add cinnamon, nutmeg, cardamom, and cloves. Mix well.

5. Transfer to a bowl and serve.

6. You can use your favorite berries or fruits for decoration.

Donuts

Ingredients:

- 1/2 cup coconut milk
- 20 drops of red food coloring
- A pinch of salt
- 1 tbsp. cocoa powder
- 1/2 cup Erythritol
- 1/2 cup flaxseed meal
- 2 cup almond flour
- 1 tsp. baking powder
- 1 tsp. vanilla extract
- 2 eggs
- 3 tbsp. coconut oil

Preparations:

1. In a bowl, mix almond flour, flaxseed meal, cocoa powder, baking powder, salt, and erythritol.

2. In another bowl, mix coconut oil with fresh coconut milk, vanilla extract, food coloring, eggs, and stir.

3. Combine 2 mixtures and stir using a hand mixer.

4. Transfer to a piping bag and shape 12 donuts on a baking sheet.

5. Place in an oven at 350F and bake for 10 to 15 minutes. Serve.

Keto Blueberry Smoothie

Ingredients:

- 1 tsp. vanilla extract

- 1 tsp. MCT or coconut oil

- 30 g protein powder

- 1 cup coconut or almond milk

- 1/2 cup blueberries

Preparations:

1. Put everything in a blender and blend until smooth.

Slow Cooker Pizza

Ingredients:

- 1 teaspoon garlic powder

- Salt and pepper to taste

- 14-ounces no-sugar-added pasta sauce

- 2 cups shredded mozzarella

- 2 cups shredded cheddar cheese

Preparations:

1. Heat a skillet.
2. Add meat, garlic, salt, and pepper.
3. When meat is no longer brown, drain any excess grease.
4. Grease your slow cooker with a coconut oil-based spray.
5. Add beef to the bottom, then add sauce and cheese on top.
6. Close the lid.
7. Cook on low for 4 hours. Enjoy!

Holiday Lamb W/ Mint + Asparagus

Ingredients:

- 2 tablespoons grass-fed butter
- 1 teaspoon dried parsley
- 1 teaspoon dried thyme
- Salt and pepper to taste
- 5 cups fresh asparagus
- 3 minced garlic cloves
- 1/2 cup fresh chopped mint
- 1/2 cup water

Preparations:

1. Dry the lamb and season with salt, pepper, parsley, and thyme.
2. Add butter to a large skillet and heat.
3. Add lamb to sear on both sides, about 2 to 5 minutes per side.
4. Put the lamb in the slow cooker.
5. Add mint and garlic.

6. Pour in water. Close the lid. Cook for 10 hours on low.
7. When that Times up, remove lamb.
8. Put asparagus in your slow cooker, then return lamb on top of the veggies.
9. Close the lid and cook for 2 hours. Serve!

Spinach-Lamb Curry

Ingredients:

- 2 tablespoons minced fresh ginger

- 2 teaspoons cumin

- 2 teaspoons gram masala

- Salt to taste

- 1 pound fresh spinach

- One 14.5 ounce can of tomatoes

- 1 chopped onion

- 2 minced garlic cloves

Preparations:

1. Put everything in your slow cooker and stir.
2. Close the lid.
3. Cook overnight for 8 hours on low.
4. Taste and season with salt if necessary!

Easy Shredded Taco Pork

Ingredients:

- 1/2 teaspoon crushed red pepper flakes

- Drizzle of extra-virgin olive oil

- Salt and pepper to taste

- 1 cup chicken stock

- 2 tablespoons chili powder

- 2 teaspoons ground cumin

- 1 teaspoon ground garlic

Preparations:

1. Mix your dry spices in a bowl.
2. Rub the oil into pork, and then spices, so they stick better.
3. Marinate for at least 1 hour in the fridge.
1. When it "s Timeto cook, add stock to your slow cooker and put in the meat.
4. Cook for 2 to 6 hours on low.

Pork Adobo Tacos

Ingredients:

- Salt and pepper to taste

- Water

- 8 low-carb tortillas

- 3 large chopped tomatoes

- 8 large lettuce leaves

- 5 minced garlic cloves

- 2 chipotle peppers in adobo sauce)

- 2 dried ancho chili peppers

- 1 chopped onion

- 1 tablespoon coriander

- 1 teaspoon paprika

- 1 teaspoon dried oregano

Preparations:

1. Heat a skillet and add both ancho chili peppers.

2. After 3-5 minutes, remove from the heat and cool.
3. Remove the seeds and chop.
4. Add chilies to a pot and pour in water, so they "recovered.
5. Bring to a boil, then reduce the heat to simmer for just 5 minutes.
6. Turn off the burner and wait 30 minutes, so peppers infuse the water.
7. When that Times up, pour into a blender with chipotle peppers, seasonings, garlic, and onion.
8. Blend well to make your adobo sauce.
9. Pat pork dry and season well with salt and pepper.
10. Spoon some adobo sauce into the cooker to coat the bottom.
11. Add pork and pour in the rest of the sauce.
12. Close the lid.
13. Cook on low for 6-8 hours.

14. To serve, shred in the sauce and serve with low-carb tortillas, chopped tomatoes, and lettuce.

Ribs Homemade Sauce

Ingredients:

- 1 teaspoon onion powder

- 1 teaspoon garlic powder

- 1 teaspoon cumin

- Salt and pepper to taste

- Enough homemade BBQ sauce to cover ribs*

- BBQ sauce can be found in the "Condiments" chapter

Preparations:

1. Mix dry seasonings in a bowl.
2. Rub into the ribs.
3. Pour BBQ sauce into your slow cooker.
4. Add ribs, turning to coat in the sauce.
5. Close the lid.
6. Cook on low for 10-12 hours.
7. When Times up, remove the ribs and put on a parchment-paper-lined cookie sheet.

8. Preheat your oven broiler.

9. Brush the ribs with 1 cup sauce on one side.

10. Stick under the broiler for 2 to 3 minutes to get a little caramelization going Serve!

Pork Shoulder Gravy

Ingredients:

- 1 tablespoon extra virgin olive oil

- 1 tablespoon paprika

- 1 teaspoon cumin

- Salt and pepper to taste

- Handful of parsley

- 2 cups heavy cream

- 1 cup water

- 1 bay leaf

- 1 small chopped onion

- 2 minced garlic cloves

Preparations:

1. Pat meat dry. Rub with oil.
2. Rub on dry spices.
3. Put meat in your slow cooker and pour in water, bay leaf, onion, and garlic.

4. Cook on low for 6 to 8 hours.

5. When Times up, remove the meat and tent with foil on a plate.

6. Strain the cooking liquid and discard solids.

7. Pour into a sauce and bring to a boil.

8. Reduce heat, and cook until you get 1 cup of liquid.

9. Slowly pour the liquid into another saucepan with the cream.

10. Bring to a boil again, and then reduce for 15-20 minutes.

11. Serve pork with gravy and a handful of parsley for garnish!

Mustard-Glazed Ham

Ingredients:

- 1 tablespoon stone-ground mustard no sugar added

- 1 teaspoon Sukrin Gold brown sugar substitute

- 4 tablespoons apple cider vinegar

- 3 tablespoons water

Preparations:

1. Pour water into your slow cooker.
2. Put in the ham.
3. In a bowl, mix mustard, vinegar, and Sukrin Gold.
4. Spoon on the meatiest part of the ham and close the lid.
5. Cook on low for 5 to 7 hours. Serve!

Rum-Glazed Ham

Ingredients:

- 1 teaspoon white wine vinegar

- Pinch of cloves

- Salt to taste

- 1 cup granulated stevia

- 2 cup water

- 1 cup light rum

- 1 teaspoon ground mustard

Preparations:

1. Trim the fat from the shank.
2. To score the meat, put the ham on a cutting board with the skin facing up.
3. Cut a criss-cross pattern across the sides and top, about a half-inch deep.
4. Pour water into your slow cooker.

5. Mix the rest of the Ingredients: to make the glaze.
6. Brush all over the ham and put in your slow cooker.
7. Close the lid.
8. Cook for 4-6 hours on low.
9. Serve!

CPSIA information can be obtained
at www.ICGtesting.com
Printed in the USA
LVHW051259111121
702999LV00019B/1117

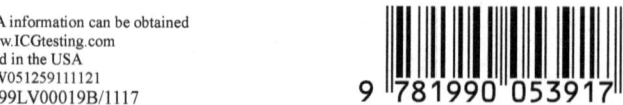